Contents

Introduction 4

THC versus CBD: Getting High versus Getting Healthy 8

How CBD Works in The Body 11

The Health Benefits of CBD 14

    What The Research is Showing 14

    Neuroprotective and Antioxidant Effects 15

    Hostile to Anxiety and Mood Enhancement 16

    Mitigating and Pain Reduction......................18

    Squeamishness, Diabetes, Epilepsy and others 20

    Psychospiritual Effects...................................21

    Quality and Potency.......................................22

Proven Health Benefits of CBD Oil......................27

    Amazing Anti-Inflammatory...........................31

    Stress and uneasiness Relief.........................33

    Diabetes Prevention......................................35

    Squeamishness..36

    Seizure Treatment...37

CBD Oil - How It's Made.......................................41

Liquor extraction. 43

CO2 extraction 44

Seasoning and weakening 46

CBD Dosage Recommendations 47

1. Lift Appetite In Cancer Patients 49

2. Straightforwardness Chronic Pain 50

3. Arrangement Relief In Epilepsy 51

4. Treat Movement Problems Associated With Huntington's Disease 52

5. Oversee Sleep Disorders 54

6. Diminish Multiple Sclerosis Symptoms 55

7. Help Manage Schizophrenia 57

8. Offer Relief In Glaucoma 57

Streamlining Your CBD Oil Dosage 59

Vaping CBD Oil? 60

Facts on CBD Oil 66

What is CBD? Precisely what is CBD Oil? 66

What's the contrast between CBD hemp oil and the hemp items I purchase at the market? 67

For what reason would it be advisable for me to utilize CBD from regular sources? 69

I heard the FDA was closing down CBD organizations. Is this valid? 70

Precisely what's the contrast among Hemp and Marijuana? 70

Are hemp inferred cannabinoids, for example, CBD as incredible as CBD from cannabis? 73

Is a standard hemp seed oil the like a high-CBD hemp separate? 75

What is CO2 extraction? What's the distinction in the middle of subcritical and supercritical CO2 extractions? 76

Precisely what is the endocannabinoid system (ECS)? 79

Introduction

CBD, generally alluded to as cannabidiol, can be drawn out from the hemp or cannabis plants. A huge number of research thinks about performed in the course of the most recent couple of years are uncovering that CBD may have a vast scope of recuperating points of interest, albeit more research is required.

It's difficult to switch on the news nowadays without hearing reports of cannabis and hemp being sanctioned far and wide - and with incredible reason: these 2 plants have been essential to mankind as prescriptions, nourishment, fuel, fiber and more for incalculable years. They're especially sheltered, develop very and consummately in numerous atmospheres, and have an uncommon rundown of valuable uses. It's as though Mother Nature created them just for us.

Furthermore, as a general rule, that is not an amazingly fantastical idea. The body really contains extraordinary receptors all through the nerve framework that are explicitly activated by substances found basically in the cannabis and hemp plants. Like, for example, CBD (Cannabidiol), a fringe wonderful aggravate that is by and by being vigorously researched far and wide and is uncovering promising signs as a potential treatment for some significant ailments in both creature and human models, notwithstanding an all out wellbeing protectant and sponsor.

Despite the fact that it's too soon to make any authoritative wellbeing claims with respect to precisely what CBD can or can't do, the examination around the substance is utilizing a look into potential mending utilizes, some of which we'll investigate beneath, and episodic reports from huge quantities of individuals around the globe program that without a doubt there is something one of a kind about CBD oil.

Inning understanding with Nora Volkow, the chief of the National Institute on Drug Abuse, "Thorough logical examinations are as yet expected to assess the therapeutic capability of CBD for explicit conditions. All things considered, pre-clinical research (comprising of both cell culture and creature plans) has really uncovered CBD to have a progression of effects that might be remedially useful, including against seizure, cancer prevention agent, neuroprotective, mitigating, pain relieving, hostile to tumor, against insane, and against nervousness properties."

Evidently Cannabidiol has a great deal taking the plunge. The street ahead will incorporate twofold visually impaired human clinical preliminaries to check or deny these early discoveries that certainly show up amazingly engaging. Nonetheless, meanwhile, that has not halted

wellbeing searchers worldwide from taking in
CBD with the expectation that they may exploit
its alleged impacts - and various are revealing
positive encounters in accordance with precisely
what the analysts are finding.

THC versus CBD: Getting High versus Getting Healthy

Specialists have really found out about CBD for quite a while, more than 60 years to be careful, anyway have very disregarded it for its a lot hotter and stunning cousin, THC, which is the essential dynamic fixing in maryjane (weed) responsible for the "high" individuals experience when smoking it.

Be that as it may, as investigation into the plant progressed during the 1970s, scientists began to examine CBD's favorable circumstances all the more intently and perceived that it was similarly as urgent as THC, if not more so in various strategies. What's more, furthermore, CBD was non-psychoactive, implying that it doesn't get you high.

Thus, CBD oil is lawful in every one of the 50 U.S. states and in most of areas everywhere throughout the world (as long as the cbd oil is separated from the hemp plant and not maryjane). A phenomenal method to consider it is THC gets you high and CBD does not. The 2 relate yet absolutely different substances existing in both the cannabis (weed) and hemp plants.

They both work freely of one another and synergistically together to create recuperating and wellbeing in the brain and body, be that as it may, CBD oil just makes you feel superb - with no sort of inebriating high.

Remember: THC is simply present in critical amounts in cannabis - likewise alluded to as weed. The hemp plant, which stays in precisely the same family as cannabis, anyway is a totally different plant, just comprises of follow amounts of THC. So smidgen, in actuality, that hemp items are totally legitimate everywhere throughout the United States and in a great deal of parts of the world.

Hemp similarly contains rates of Cannabidiol that can be expanded by uncommon rearing practices, through centering the CBD normally found in hemp oil and using conventional plant-extraction systems.

How CBD Works in The Body

In contrast to THC, CBD is particular in that it has a wide assortment of effects on some of the body's vital frameworks that are in charge of controling our wellbeing. CBD has a liking for activating serotonin receptors (explicitly 5-HT1A), which control pressure and nervousness, serenity and perspective; vanilloid receptors, which oversee and direct how we experience torment; adenosine receptors, which deal with the quality and profundity of our rest; and in a roundabout way impacts endocannabinoid receptors, which control memory, vitality levels, feelings of anxiety, inconvenience resistance, body temperature level and craving, among numerous others things.

CBD: Learn About the Extraordinay Health Benefits of CBD Oilcounter clockwise from upper left: CBD rich maryjane bud, THC precious stones,

CBD bottomless hemp oil, CBD extricate gum. Cannabidiol itself is non-psychoactive in spite of the fact that it very well may be extricated from the (cannabis plant). financially offered, legitimate CBD things, be that as it may, are for the most part extricated from hemp oil.

Researchers have entirely found in theoretical creature and human cell culture plans (importance that they are uncovering human and creature cells to various convergences of CBD in petri dishes and test tubes in the lab) that CBD has hostile to tumor impacts on glioma and bosom carcinomas and results in expanded disease cell demise in explicit sorts of malignant growths.

As it at present stands, it's a tremendous jump from the test cylinder to the human body, and no conclusive cases can be made in such manner, anyway loads of in theclinical neighborhood are viewing these improvements incredibly cautiously.

In that capacity, it keeps on being examined cautiously as a conceivable 'wonder medicate' by both nutraceutical and pharmaceutical organizations around the world. Every day it appears to be a pristine research contemplate is being propelled affirming or singing the praises of another assortment of addition from CBD, which is being hailed in various clinical circles as a standout amongst the most astounding fresh out of the box new prescriptions found in decades.

The Health Benefits of CBD

What The Research is Showing

So just precisely what is so incredible about CBD oil's advantages that is causing a ton intrigue and research in both the logical and therapeutic networks? To comprehend that effectively, it's critical to see how CBD functions in the psyche and body.

Neuroprotective and Antioxidant Effects

Of all CBD's archived outcomes a standout amongst its most novel and fascinating is neuroprotection, which is thought to originate from its ability to work as an incredible cell reinforcement in the cerebrum.

Neuroprotection freely alludes to the capacity of Cannabidiol- - as appeared in an assortment of creature contemplates - to a) counteract, moderate, turn around or disturb some of the methodology that outcome in the breakdown of nerve cells in the cerebrum and sensory system thought to cause numerous normal illnesses as alzheimer Parkinson's, MS, strokes and that's only the tip of the iceberg, and b) limit swelling in the mind, which is thought by various specialists to ruin cerebrum work and contribute covertly ailments like ceaseless tiredness and mind haze.

Albeit neuroprotective effects have very just been appeared creature models and cell societies, there is trust that CBD may apply comparable effects in people, however more research is required.

Hostile to Anxiety and Mood Enhancement

A standout amongst the most detectable outcomes that bunches of individuals report in the wake of taking CBD oil is a lovely and incredible decrease in pressure and tension and a noticeable lift in perspective. Bunches of clarify feeling an influx of quiet and joy washing over their bodies, which pursues CBD's accounted for results at 5-HT receptors that deal with the arrival of loads of fundamental synapses that influence pressure/tension dimensions and state of mind, especially serotonin.

One investigation of CBD separate on nervousness utilized practical attractive reverberation imaging (fMRI), which is a propelled cerebrum action mapping instrument, to think about what jumped out at the mind when people took 600mg of CBD extricate while being presented to pressure and uneasiness actuating boosts. What they found was that CBD loosened up the amygdala and cingulate cortex, 2 urgent areas of the cerebrum mainstream to oversee dread, strain levels and stress and tension, to give some examples things.

In another exploration examine, Brazilian researchers examined the consequence of CBD separate on human cortisol levels in eleven volunteers. They found that CBD diminished cortisol levels essentially more than the fake treatment which most subjects moreover detailed a soothing impact from the treatment.

In a meta-examination of CBD's effects on tension performed in Brazil, researchers found that "contemplates using creature plans of uneasiness and including sound volunteers evidently prescribe an anxiolytic-like aftereffect of CBD. Furthermore,

Cannabidiol extricate was uncovered to diminish uneasiness in patients with social tension issue."

Therefore, CBD is likewise being explored as a characteristic stimulant, hostile to insane, and a choice to SSRI meds (Prozac, and so on.).

Mitigating and Pain Reduction

Different creature considers have demonstrated that CBD has an astounding capacity to diminish explicit cell forms that bring about swelling and, accordingly, torment.

Researchers are right now completing exploration concentrates to see exactly how much this effect exchanges over to people, anyway there have really been various logical preliminaries in Europe on an item called Sativex, which is a 1:1 blend of CBD and THC.

These exploration examines found that Sativex had the capacity to bring down agony identified with focal and fringe neuropathy, rheumatoid joint inflammation, and malignant growth to changing degrees in a large portion of the examination members. It is hazy exactly the amount of an outcome Cannabidiol has on torment decline in these cases, in any case, the creature thinks about propose that CBD is likely included somewhat dependent on its perceived effects on cell forms.

In spite of the fact that the jury is still out about how powerful CBD oils and concentrates are for swelling, loads of who have been fighting with irritation related sickness like joint pain have detailed that CBD oils, concentrates and creams comprising of CBD have really helped in diminishing a couple of their signs.

Squeamishness, Diabetes, Epilepsy and others

Despite the fact that not as run of the mill, considers on creatures and a couple of, little human investigations (on account of epilepsy) moreover discovered that Cannabidiol indicates vow as a potential treatment for seizures, diabetes and queasiness, to give some examples things, albeit more research ponder is required.

Three of the 4 human investigations done using CBD as a treatment for epilepsy indicated positive results, by and by, due to make blemishes and nonattendance of meticulousness, numerous researchers are recommending that the at present promptly accessible data is deficient to reach firm determinations seeing the viability of CBD as a treatment for seizures.

Studies are at present in progress to get much better information dependent on primer engaging lead to creature preliminaries.

Psychospiritual Effects

While the psychospiritual impacts of (weed) are amazing, CBD is a later, less usually used compound, along these lines its effects and favorable circumstances in this area aren't totally seen yet. So, as referenced beforehand, many feel a stamped sedation and even sentiments of satisfaction or broad unwinding in the wake of expending top quality CBD oils and concentrates.

All things considered, CBD oil is often used by meditators to "go further, faster" as it can help with a couple of the psychological babble that much of the time surfaces amid training. Others report that the surprising, positive move in outlook that CBD oil can create is valuable in observing life from an alternate perspective that multiple occasions fits new experiences, thoughts, and conclusion about things that some time ago disturbed them.

Quality and Potency

More so than different herbs and plants, quality can be a worry with specific CBD items, so it's imperative to search out brands with a high level of security that unmistakably disclose their sourcing practices and quality principles. Search for things that are totally characteristic or possibly contain natural CBD as these are guaranteed to be without harming synthetic compounds and solvents that are frequently used in the extraction methodology of less-trustworthy organizations simply out to make a buck.

All usually offered, lawful CBD things are extricated from the hemp plant, and especially hemp oil, though items that are legitimate in certain spots however unlawful in others (contingent upon local purview) are frequently drawn out from weed (cannabis) plants and incorporate extensive and shifting dimensions of THC.

There is some proof that rates of THC increment the proficiency of CBD, in any case, it isn't required to receive the rewards of taking Cannabidiol. Research think about has uncovered unadulterated CBD removes from hemp and hemp oil, as long as the CBD is of high caliber, are likewise effective and helpful. In any case, in progressively genuine, relentless medical issues there might be extra advantages from having THC in the blend, for example, increasingly articulated uneasiness decline and therapeutic effects, inning agreement with the diverse human investigations did on the substance.

It is similarly critical to consider quality while choosing CBD things as well. Generally, the impacts of CBD are portion dependent somewhat, proposing that the more that is devoured, the more articulated its outcomes are. In that capacity, it's basic to search for increasingly focused and additionally very absorbable things for ideal impact. There are a wide assortment of Cannabidiol item potencies promptly accessible, yet an extraordinary beginning stage for most of individuals is for one measurement of the thing to be in the 2mg to 7mg assortment, with the last being on the more dominant side.

On the off chance that you realize you will in general be sensitive to characteristic items and prescriptions, start at a lower portion. On the off chance that you don't tend to feel anything or comprehend you need a more grounded item to see the benefits of CBD, don't hesitate regardless higher measurements. For some CBD hemp oil things, you can take an incomplete or twofold measurement to alter the adequacy.

CBD oil is strikingly protected and has uncovered itself to be sensibly symptom free so there's nothing to worry over except if you have a known unfavorably susceptible response to hemp or you are on some sort of medicine or therapeutic supervision. If all else fails look for guidance from an affirmed naturopath or doctor. As usual, when starting new herbs or characteristic drugs like Cannabidiol, influence sure to start moderate to fathom how your body reacts and create to higher doses after some time.

Proven Health Benefits of CBD Oil

California was the absolute first state to approve medicinal cannabis in 1996. From that point forward, 27 additional states and Washington, D.C., have really authorized its restorative use.

What's more, after the November 2016 decision, the Golden State went into the 25% of the nation that likewise approaches lawful relaxation pot.

This "green dash for unheard of wealth" is among the best financial patterns today. What's more, it's just a question of time before cannabis use is authorized in some sort the nation over.

California without a doubt started a development on the restorative cannabis front. One where doctors could exhort it as a treatment for seizures, malignant growth, joint pain, ceaseless inconvenience, HIV/AIDS, epilepsy, numerous sclerosis, headaches, resting scatters, nervousness, PTSD, diminished craving and then some.

Research ponders demonstrate that the medicinal favorable circumstances of cannabis are certain. Which's gratitude to substances inside the plant called cannabinoids.

There are in excess of 60 sorts of cannabinoids in maryjane. THC is the most-discussed, as this is the one that offers the hallucinogenic outcomes.

Be that as it may, on the off chance that you don't approach cannabis ... or then again wish to keep away from any of its possibly cerebrum modifying impacts

Give me a chance to introduce you to a different - and legitimate - compound.

It's called cannabidiol, or CBD for short.

CBD is the huge non-psychoactive component of Cannabis sativa. (The clinical term for a sort of cannabis.).

As per a 2013 research examine distributed in the British Journal of Clinical Pharmacology, CBD works as an:.

- Calming.

- Anticonvulsant (or, hostile to seizure agent).

- Cancer prevention agent.

- Antiemetic (agent versus queasiness, development affliction and hurling). Anxiolytic (tension reducer), and.

- Antipsychotic specialist.

just to give some examples...

What's more, CBD oil is totally legitimate because of the way that it very well may be drawn out from hemp, a nearby cousin of cannabis.

Presently, hemp isn't generally legitimate to develop in each U.S. state. Anyway the Food and Drug Administration records CBD oil as a "dietary enhancement." That shows you can get it on the web and have it given to any state.

Amazing Anti-Inflammatory.

I've created to you in many cases about the threats of agony relievers and non-steroidal enemy of inflammatories like Tylenol and Advil.

Standard medications like these can accompany serious physical reactions like ulcers, liver harm and inner dying.

Also, sedative based painkillers like Vicodin and hydrocodone are huge elements to the considerably more-perilous compulsion scourge our nation manages.

Industrious swelling has been connected to disease like malignant growth, heart issue, diabetes, rheumatoid joint pain, neurodegenerative scatters like Alzheimer's, and bunches of others.

In case you're hunting down an option in contrast to the hazardous pharmaceuticals used to treat these kind of conditions, look close to CBD oil.

Studies have really indicated CBD significantly smothers perpetual incendiary and neuropathic inconvenience. What's more, it does as such without activating pain relieving (or, painkiller) resilience.

To puts it basically ...

Not at all like sedative agony relievers- - which just cover torment and quickly develop a resilience in the body- - CBD is an effective mitigating that does not lose its proficiency with time.

Stress and uneasiness Relief.

Another plague by and by destroying the U.S. is our reliance on hurtful pressure and nervousness prescriptions like Xanax, Valium and Ativan.

These are transient arrangements that bring a high danger of enslavement. However, it would appear that some therapeutic experts hand them out like Halloween treat.

CBD oil is a characteristic elective that can be similarly as dependable, without the negative antagonistic impacts.

CBD oil has really been uncovered to bring down pressure and nervousness in customers with social uneasiness condition. Analysts prescribe that it might in like manner work for fit of anxiety, over the top habitual condition, social tension issue and injury.

A 2011 research examine looked at the effects of a reenactment open talking test. Scientists checked solid control customers, and treatment-local customers with social pressure and tension condition.

An in general of 24 never-treated customers with social pressure and uneasiness condition were given either CBD or a fake treatment 1.5 hours before the test.

Researchers found that pre-treatment with CBD fundamentally decreased pressure and uneasiness, psychological incapacity and distress in their discourse productivity.

The fake treatment bunch displayed higher pressure and tension, intellectual weakness and uneasiness.

Diabetes Prevention.

Practically HALF of the U.S populace either has diabetes or uncovers pre-diabetes signs.

This dangerous ailment represents its own everyday medical issues. Anyway it in like manner puts you at a lot more serious hazard for coronary illness, kidney disappointment, nerve harm, and various different clutters.

Studies have discovered that CBD treatment extensively brings down the peril of diabetes in mice. The event dropped from 86% in non-offered mice 30% in CBD-treated mice.

Which means, CBD impactsly affects your glucose and can lessen your danger of diabetes.

Squeamishness.

CBD is a powerful squeamishness and hurling reducer, similarly as cannabis has really been advanced for a considerable length of time.

A 2012 research consider discharged in the British Journal of Pharmacology found that CBD points of interest included enemy of sickness and antiemetic impacts (trust development disease, and chemotherapy reactions) when it was directed.

Next time you're feeling somewhat woozy, don't go after the TUMS or Pepto. Consider this regular substitute rather.

Seizure Treatment.

Cannabis has uncovered on numerous occasions its capacity to manage seizures where different sorts of present day drug have really fizzled.

These exceptional impacts have really been a reviving weep for restorative cannabis supporters. This is among the main powers behind its broad (and endeavor I state "developing") legitimization.

Presently, science is uncovering CBD can give a similar sort of treatment.

For example, a 2014 Stanford University study uncovered great outcomes for the utilization of cannabidiols to treat kids with epilepsy.

A critical note: The normal number of against epileptic medications endeavored before utilizing CBD was 12.

Sixteen of the 19 mothers and fathers (84%) revealed a decrease in their tyke's seizure recurrence while taking CBD cannabis. Of these:.

Two (11%) announced total seizure adaptability.

8 (42%) announced a more noteworthy than 80% decrease in seizure recurrence.

Six (32%) detailed a 25%- - 60% seizure decline.

Other advantageous effects included expanded readiness, much better state of mind and improved rest; while negative impacts included drowsiness and weariness.

Several Other Potential Benefits

CBD has been studied for its role in treating a number of health issues other than those outlined above.

Though more studies are needed, CBD is thought to provide the following health benefits:

• Antipsychotic effects: Studies suggest that CBD may help people with schizophrenia and other mental disorders by reducing psychotic symptoms .

• Substance abuse treatment: CBD has been shown to modify circuits in the brain related to drug addiction. In rats, CBD has been shown to reduce morphine dependence and heroin-seeking behavior .

• Anti-tumor effects: In test-tube and animal studies, CBD has demonstrated anti-tumor effects. In animals, it has been shown to prevent the spread of breast, prostate, brain, colon and lung cancer.

• Diabetes prevention: In diabetic mice, treatment with CBD reduced the incidence of diabetes by 56% and significantly reduced inflammation .

CBD Oil - How It's Made

CBD oil overwhelmed the world a few years back when Dr. Sanjay Gupta inspected the cannabinoid's capacity to treat kids with epilepsy.

At first, CBD oil was considered as a medication for the fundamentally sick. Of late, it has picked up fame with the overall population as it's advantages are getting to be known.

As a buyer of CBD oils, it is basic for you to know how they are made.

Creating top quality CBD oil starts with picking the appropriate weed hereditary qualities. Regardless of whether you are creating oil from cannabis or hemp plants, choosing a strain that is normally high in CBD is vital.

The present well known CBD makers have worked for quite a long time to create exclusive groups of cannabis plants. While you can remove CBD from numerous cannabis strains, choosing an innate that is normally high in CBD will build yields and quality.

When the developing method is done, the plant material is set for extraction.

There are a scope of CBD oil items on the commercial center. A couple of them are "entire plant" removes. Others are detached concentrates.

Whole plant proposes essentially precisely what you figure it does- - the entire plant is used for extraction. This methodology is famous in the medicinal networks because of the way that it is trusted that a more extensive range of cannabinoids is recorded amid extraction.

The cannabinoid range is fundamental since it spurs the "company result", which invigorates the endocannabinoid framework.

There are likewise CBD confines that are "unadulterated" CBD. These confines depend totally on the viability of the CBD and at last the nature of the qualities used to get it.

Liquor extraction.

Entire plant CBD oils can be made in an assortment of techniques. The "underlying" CBD oil was created by Rick Simpson. With this methodology you splash the plant material in a dissolvable, for example, grain liquor. When the item drenches, the staying fluid is brimming with CBD (and different cannabinoids), you vanish the dissolvable and the staying oil is prepared for use.

The Rick Simpson approach impacted greater activities to scale their extraction for business request. Today, ethanol is usually used to extricate CBD for oils. This technique expects you to splash the plant item in ethanol and after that the subsequent liquor administration is executed by means of "Roto-Vap".

The Roto-Vap warms the liquor, making it vaporize. Rather than vaporizing into the air, the Roto-Vap recovers the ethanol for later use. In a different chamber, the CBD oil is sans left of the dissolvable and prepared for admission.

CO_2 extraction

Another well known way to deal with draw out CBD from cannabis is with CO_2. This strategy requires more aptitude and unquestionably a larger number of gadgets than the liquor procedure. CO_2 extraction requires a progression of chambers that control temperature level and weight.

The temperature level and weight in the chambers trigger the CO_2 in the cannabinoids to react and isolate. As the cannabinoids fluctuate, they are assembled in various chambers. This system allows an extractor to isolate the cannabinoids and in the end acquaint only those favored with their dish.

These are by all account not the only systems for illustration out CBD from cannabis, yet they are surely the most prevalent today. Be that as it may, drawing out CBD is just piece of making CBD oil.

Seasoning and weakening

The drawn out oil is commonly not the best tasting. Since clients are expecting to utilize CBD oils as a day by day part of their lives, makers are attempting to make their things tasty.

Also, clients need different qualities of CBD, so makers should "weaken" their crude CBD oils to suit.

As a purchaser of CBD things, you have to concentrate first on where the plant item utilized for generation is sourced. The absolute best organizations in the CBD oil advertise are vertically fused, giving control of value and wellbeing from seed to deal.

CBD Dosage Recommendations

The appropriate measure of CBD can help transform you

An essential CBD oil portion works amazing for general wellbeing. In any case, for the individuals who have serious conditions, as well as can be expected give a whole fresh out of the plastic new rent on your wellbeing.

CBD (cannabidiol) is a plant compound found in hemp. Through different extraction systems, CBD is sourced from hemp plants and stalks to build up an oil that utilizes enormous medical advantages. Whenever devoured, CBD follows up on the body's endocannabinoid framework (ECS) to advance homeostasis.

Normally taking the base prescribed portion of CBD (we propose 4 drops, multiple times day with our Superior CBD, for a generally speaking of 1 ml) utilizes in general prosperity to adjust the nerve framework, advance mental clearness, help sound aggravation response, and give propelled cancer prevention agent support.

For those with specific wellbeing sicknesses, an expanded CBD oil portion is expected to supply alleviation.

Inning agreement with CannLabs, the nation's driving full-administration testing lab for cannabis items, there is no perceived deadly CBD measurement.

The truth of the matter is, it's difficult to overdose on CBD. The National Cancer Institute states, "In light of the fact that cannabinoid receptors, not at all like narcotic receptors, are not arranged in the cerebrum stem areas controlling breath, fatal overdoses from Cannabis and cannabinoids don't occur."

1. Lift Appetite In Cancer Patients

With disease rates developing, so are the dangers of chemotherapy. For customers who use chemo "treatment" as a strategy to battle malignant growth, a lost of hunger is a commonplace unfavorable impacts. This starts from chemo harming cells and DNA, activating queasiness, outrageous retching, low vitality, and the ECS to decrease craving. CBD advances craving and gives malignancy patients a longing to enjoy sustenance, advancing fitting sustenance and expanding the patient's munititions stockpile to battle sickness.

Perfect CBD Oil Dosage: 2.5 mg of THC by mouth with or without 1 mg of CBD day by day for about a month and a half

2. Straightforwardness Chronic Pain

In excess of 100 million Americans battle with industrious uneasiness, all begin for different reasons. Inconvenience can show in joints, muscles, organs, body pits, bones, and tendons; here and there set off by infections, for example, Crohn's, ulcerative colitis, Lyme illness, a few sclerosis, and fibromyalgia.

Relentless sickness can be devastating and the related torment can leave customers immobilized and powerless to work when flare-ups occur. Research contemplate demonstrates that CBD can bolster solid joint, muscle, and organ work and bring distress alleviation. By following up on the ECS, CBD impacts nociceptive ways to altogether decrease swelling- - a main purpose behind ailment and ceaseless agony - and avoid torment.

Ideal CBD Oil Dosage: Sublingual ingestion of 2.5-20 mg CBD for a normal of 25 days. Advantages are combined.

3. Arrangement Relief In Epilepsy

In 2015, an investigation in American Academy of Neurology offered the lab aftereffects of 137 seizure exploited people who used the FDA approved medication Epidiolex—a pharmaceutical oil-based concentrate of CBD. Ages went from two to 26 and provided the rundown beneath results:

Seizures diminished by around 54 percent in 137 people who finished 12 weeks on Epidiolex.

Customers who had Dravet Syndrome (DS) responded all the more emphatically with a 63 percent diminishing in seizures more than 3 months

In 27 patients with atonic seizures (which are much of the time found in people with Lennox-Gastaut Syndrome (LGS) alongside different kinds of epilepsy), the atonic seizures decreased by 66.7 percent generally.

Ideal CBD Oil Dosage: Sublingual admission of 200-300 mg of CBD day by day for up to 4 1/2 months.

4. Treat Movement Problems Associated With Huntington's Disease

Huntington's illness is an obtained focal sensory system condition that triggers a degeneration of nerve cells in the mind. Poor coordination, negligible capacity abilities, and jerky, irregular, and wild movements win side effects.

Through following up on CB1 and CB2 receptors, CBD moderates the movement of neurodegeneration in Huntington's ailment. This is accomplished by limiting lethality in microglial cells and stifling irritation to advance helpful alleviation in joints and muscles. This eases hyper-active signs and functions as a neuro

This is accomplished by limiting poisonous quality in microglial cells and stifling irritation to advance remedial alleviation in joints and muscles. This reduces hyper-dynamic signs and fills in as a neuroprotector in degenerative sicknesses like Huntington's disease.

CBD Dosage Recommendation: Sublingual admission of 10 mg of CBD per 1 lb of weight, day by day for about a month and a half

5. Oversee Sleep Disorders

Americans balance 6.9 hours a rest each night. Join that with an inability to rest all through the daytime because of work, long drives, reliable blue lights from when we wake until we drop off to lay down with our telephones in our grasp, and we're inclining towards a wellbeing disaster. Rest issue change from dozing issue - 70 million exploited people in the only us, narcolepsy, obstructive rest apnea, and delayed rest organize disorder.

Research uncovers CBD to be proficient in treating rest related concerns. A recent report demonstrated CBD's capacity to bring down migraines in military laborers experiencing PTSD. CBD's ability to follow up on the ECS may enable it to work with the body's natural beat moreover.

In like manner, one research examine demonstrated that when CBD was taken in with the lights on, it viably expanded readiness - all around expected to dispose of indications of lack of sleep. Another exploration think about in 2013 uncovered that CBD had the capacity to build generally speaking rest time in grown-up male rodents amid the evening time.

Ideal CBD Oil Dosage: Sublingual ingestion of 40-160 mg of CBD day by day

6. Diminish Multiple Sclerosis Symptoms

A few Sclerosis is a neurodegenerative immune system malady that influences the cerebrum, spinal string, and optic nerve. This causes a wide range of medical issues comprising of vision misfortune, industrious torment, exhaustion, and debilitated coordination.

Mixes like non-psychoactive CBD shut down the resistant framework, halting the vicious assault on the primary nerve framework. At the point when the body resistant framework is quieted down, it not assaults your fundamental nerve framework.

Ideal CBD Oil Dosage: Cannabis plant extricates comprising of 2.5-120 mg of a THC-CBD mix by mouth day by day for 2-15 weeks. An oral splash may contain 2.7 mg of THC and 2.5 mg of CBD at dosages of 2.5-120 mg for as much as about two months. Customers

typically utilize eight showers inside any 3 hours, with a limit of 48 splashes in any 24-hour length.

7. Help Manage Schizophrenia

Schizophrenia is an outrageous mental turmoil that upsets reliable discernment, correspondence, and the outflow of feeling. Research recommends CBD utilizes hostile to crazy impacts since it triggers the CB2 receptors of the ECS. This adjusts the's body invulnerable framework, bringing down and altogether diminishing insane side effects.

Perfect CBD Oil Dosage: Sublingual utilization of 40-1,280 mg CBD every day, for as much as about a month

8. Offer Relief In Glaucoma

Glaucoma happens when liquid collection in the front of the eye, expanding eye weight and hurting the optic nerve. More than three million

Americans have glaucoma, with just HALF mindful of their condition.

A recent report prescribes the neuroprotection CBD offers diminishes the quality of peroxynitrite-- a particle that can harm atoms in cells, comprising of DNA, and proteins and a specialist that causes glaucoma.

Perfect CBD Oil Dosage: Sublingual ingestion of a solitary measurement of 20-40 mg under the tongue. Measurements higher than 40 mg may really expand eye weight.

Streamlining Your CBD Oil Dosage

Shoppers must look at thing embeds completely to guarantee they are taking the perfect measure of CBD, and converse with the endorsing specialist about any worries or issues.

Vaping CBD Oil?

CBD oil has a few distinctive conveyance strategies. It is for the most part ingested, yet there's numerous other alternative

This has never been all the more genuine for cannabidiol (CBD). With the rising interest for CBD items, there are a wide range of strategies to get your ordinary measurements.

They change from sublingual splashes, to vaping CBD oils, to smoking cigarettes magnificent antiquated joints. However numerous individuals don't have a clue about that the technique which you ingest CBD can significantly change its productive measurements.

CBD's Bioavailability: Understanding Its Variations

In essential, not all the CBD you take in will straight influence your body: only a particular bit will be able to enter your foundational stream and produce its dynamic effects.

This rate is depicted in science as "bioavailability," and it exceedingly relies upon the way where CBD is exhibited to your framework. For instance, the oral bioavailability of CBD is approximately 15 percent. That suggests for each and every 100 milligrams of CBD that you eat, only 15 milligrams will truly achieve your circulatory system.

There are two principle reasons why this happens. At first, CBD is hydrophobic, implying that it isn't very water-solvent. In precisely the same strategy that oil dislikes to consolidate with vinegar, CBD dislikes to remain in your circulatory system.

Rather, it quickly diffuses from your blood and gathers into your greasy tissues. Unfortunately, this extensively limits the measure of bioactive CBD that can enter your foundational course, taking into consideration less CBD to be conveyed to its dynamic sites in your body and along these lines bringing down its complete bioavailability.

Second, when a natural substance like CBD enters your gut, it needs to experience the liver before it enters your blood course.

Amid this progress, the liver will effectively bring down the amount of CBD, either through assimilation or through substance breakdown by liver chemicals.

This marvel is known as the "main pass result," where experiencing the liver reductions the centralization of bioactive mixes.

There are several different approaches to counterbalance these misfortunes of CBD. For one, you can limit the measure of CBD that liquifies out of your circulation system by putting the CBD into a caring that is increasingly hydrophilic, or water-dissolvable.

Be that as it may, this must be accomplished by complex concoction demonstrates, for example, using cyclodextrins or liposomes. A progressively helpful choice is to sidestep the main pass consequence of oral organization totally by utilizing vaporization.

All through vaporization, CBD enters your lungs and diffuses specifically into your circulatory system as opposed to going through your gut and liver.

This stays away from the primary pass result inside and out, allowing right around 4 fold the amount of CBD to enter your stream for a most extreme bioavailability of roughly 50 to 60 percent. Basically, this infers you can achieve precisely the same useful contacts with an a lot littler measure of CBD.

Not just that, anyway vaping will impressively diminish the amount of time it thinks about the CBD in your body to end up dynamic, given that you don't have to anticipate it to go through your gut.

By vaporizing a CBD e-fluid or high-CBD concentrate, you may perhaps feel its effects 30 to a hour snappier. This makes vaping CBD an incredibly effective conveyance system.

Normally, in case you're inclining to tolerating the vape life, ensure you've done your exploration contemplate on the concentrate you plan to take in.

Without adequate regulative oversight in the developing vape and maryjane markets, couple of business have had the capacity to create an unmistakable and homogenous CBD administration, so the milligram sum in CBD things is frequently unpredictable with the amount guaranteed on the name.

Make a point to request both inside and outsider test results from your picked source to ensure you're getting a quality item!

Facts on CBD Oil

What is CBD? Precisely what is CBD Oil?

Cannabidiol (CBD) is a normally occurring constituent of business hemp/cannabis. Its equation is $C_{21}H_{30}O_2$ and it has an atomic mass of 314.4636. It is the most bottomless non-psychoactive cannabinoid found in pot, and is by and large experimentally examined for various reasons.

CBD oil is a pot oil (regardless of whether got from cannabis or modern hemp, as the word maryjane is the latin sort name for both) that has huge measures of cannabidiol (CBD) included inside it. Our CBD things and concentrates are originated from business hemp, so they could be considered CBD-rich hemp oil, hemp acquired CBD oil, CBD-rich cannabis oil, or clearly "hemp separates" since they for the most part contain considerably more than just CBD.

Indeed, cannabis doesn't recommend maryjane, anyway is the family name, and general umbrella term which a wide range of cannabis and hemp fall under. The type of cannabis we use for our CBD and hemp extricates is business hemp; we don't sell cannabis.

What's the contrast between CBD hemp oil and the hemp items I purchase at the market?

Hemp items sold in stores are frequently made with hemp seed oil, which can contain just follow measures of CBD. While it has been noticed that hemp seed oil can be an extraordinary wellspring of sustenance, its negligible amount of CBD per weight makes it unfeasible as a CBD supplement.

For what reason would it be advisable for me to utilize CBD from regular sources?

Not at all like artificially made or synthetically inferred CBD, which expels the cannabinoid from whatever is left of the plant's concentrate, our CBD hemp oil is separated from the plant in a procedure that likewise pulls the majority of the plant's unsaturated fats, waxes, sugars, nutrients and minerals, and terpenes and flavonoids, alongside the different cannabinoids present, for a progressively total dietary enhancement.

Regularly called the "escort impact", this strategy for utilizing CBD exploits the entire plant, giving the body a chance to interface with the hemp in its normal state.

Engineered CBD is additionally a controlled substance in the United States.

I heard the FDA was closing down CBD organizations. Is this valid?

The FDA has cautioned organizations showcasing CBD items not to make any cases about the utilization of CBD to treat or forestall illness. This is because of the way that the FDA has not affirmed CBD or some other cannabinoid for any restorative signs and does not presently see it as having therapeutic advantage.

Precisely what's the contrast among Hemp and Marijuana?

Logically, mechanical Hemp and Marijuana are precisely the same plant, with a sort and animal groups name of Cannabis Sativa. They have a radically different genetic profile however. Mechanical Hemp is continually a worry of Cannabis sativa, while weed can be Cannabis sativa, Cannabis indica, or Cannabis ruderalis. The huge refinement is the means by which business hemp has really been recreated contrasted and a weed type of Cannabis sativa.

As a rule, mechanical hemp is extremely stringy, with long solid stalks, and barely has any blossoming buds, while a weed weight of Cannabis sativa will be littler estimated, bushier, and loaded up with sprouting buds. Be that as it may, later modern hemp extends in the USA are being reproduced to have more blooms and more prominent yields of cannabinoids and terpenes, for example, our Kentucky hemp we're currently using!

99% of the time weed has a high measure of THC and only an actually low amount of CBD. Hemp, then again, normally has an actually high amount of CBD by and large, and just a follow measure of THC. Fortunately, the cannabinoid profile of hemp is perfect for individuals endeavoring to discover exploit cannabis without the 'high.'

Hemp is used for making natural enhancements, sustenance, fiber, rope, paper, blocks, oil, normal plastic, thus much more, while cannabis is commonly utilized essentially recreationally, profoundly, and therapeutically. The term weed oil can portray either a maryjane or hemp acquired oil, since cannabis and hemp are 2 different sorts of weed.

In the USA the legitimate meaning of "business hemp," per Section 7606 of the Agricultural Appropriations Act of 2014, is "Mechanical HEMP–The expression "modern hemp" shows the plant Cannabis sativa L. also, any piece of such plant, in the case of developing or not, with a delta-9 tetrahydrocannabinol centralization of not more than 0.3 percent on a dry weight premise."

Are hemp inferred cannabinoids, for example, CBD as incredible as CBD from cannabis?

The short reaction is yes. CBD will be CBD, regardless of whether from pot or hemp. Most of pot has a very low non-psychoactive cannabinoid profile (like CBD, CBC, CBG), so most of the time hemp would be undeniably progressively best to anything other than THC. Cannabis is generally amazingly high in THC (gives people the high) however ordinarily low in other non-psychoactive cannabinoids.

These days in the USA, heaps of ranchers are developing modern hemp blossoms that are similarly as excellent, scent delivering, and terpene rich as the absolute best weed weights, for example, our joined forces ranchers in Kentucky.

Is a standard hemp seed oil the like a high-CBD hemp separate?

In no way, shape or form. Standard hemp oil, which can be found actually reasonably at a general store, is a much different item than our CO_2 hemp extricates (not from seed). Fundamental hemp oil is created by virus squeezing the seeds, while our hemp separate is a supercritical CO_2 extraction of the hemp plant itself, not the seeds.

Hemp seed oil is pondered to be a fabulous nutritive nourishment, anyway it doesn't have the normally happening terpenes, cannabinoids and different parts that our concentrates do have.

What is CO2 extraction? What's the distinction in the middle of subcritical and supercritical CO2 extractions?

CO2 extraction is an extraction system that utilizes pressurized co2 to separate phyto-synthetics, (for example, CBD, CBG, or terpenes, flavonoids, and so on.) from a plant. CO2 at explicit temperatures and weights acts like a dissolvable, without the dangers of truly being one. It is the most costly extraction strategy, and is generally considered the most dependable and most secure plant extraction procedure on the planet.

Heaps of hemp and CBD organizations gloat about their supercritical CO2 extractions, anyway that is in reality only one (and maybe a sub-par) approach of utilizing a CO2 extraction machine. There are likewise subcritical CO2 extractions, and 'mid-basic', a fundamental range among subcritical and supercritical. Subcritical (low temperature, low weight) CO_2 extractions take additional time and produce littler estimated yields than super-basic, anyway they hold the essential oils, terpenes, and other touchy synthetic concoctions inside the plant. Supercritical, then again, is a high weight and warmth strategy that hurts most terpenes and warmth touchy synthetics, yet can extricate a lot greater particles, for example, lipids (omega 3 and 6), chlorophyll, and waxes.

A genuinely full-range CO_2 extricate comprises of absolute first playing out a subcritical extraction, isolating the drawn out oil, and after that drawing out a similar plant material utilizing super critical pressure, then homogenizing both oil extracts into one. In the vital oil industry, an extract used this specific process is described as a CO_2 Total.

Precisely what is the endocannabinoid system (ECS)?

The endocannabinoid system (ECS) is a gathering of endogenous cannabinoid receptors situated in mammalian cerebrum and all through the principle and fringe stressed frameworks, including neuromodulatory lipids and their receptors." Wikipedia.

There are 2 essential sorts of receptors in the ECS, CB1 and CB2. CB1 receptors are predominantly found in the principle nerve framework and minds of vertebrates, and CB2 are regularly found in the fringe on edge framework. There are two principle cannabinoids well evolved creatures produce-2AG and Anandamide (called after the Sanskrit expression "ananda" which means "harmony").

For a huge number of years each vertebrate on Earth has really been furnished with this ECS, a crucial framework in the body, and it has been found out about in the clinical and medicinal networks since the 1980's. In any case, it's as yet not instructed about in most therapeutic schools.

Outlook

The role of cannabidiol as a treatment for anxiety disorders remains unclear, as more long-term studies are required to assess the benefits and risks.

For people with anxiety who have gotten no relief from other treatments, however, CBD oil offers a potential alternative solution.

People considering CBD oil for anxiety should speak with a doctor to help determine the right treatment for them. People are also advised to research the laws in their area regarding the use of cannabis products.

Made in the USA
Las Vegas, NV
29 April 2022